DRUG INTERACTIONS:

PROTECTING YOURSELF FROM DANGEROUS DRUG, MEDICATION, AND FOOD COMBINATIONS

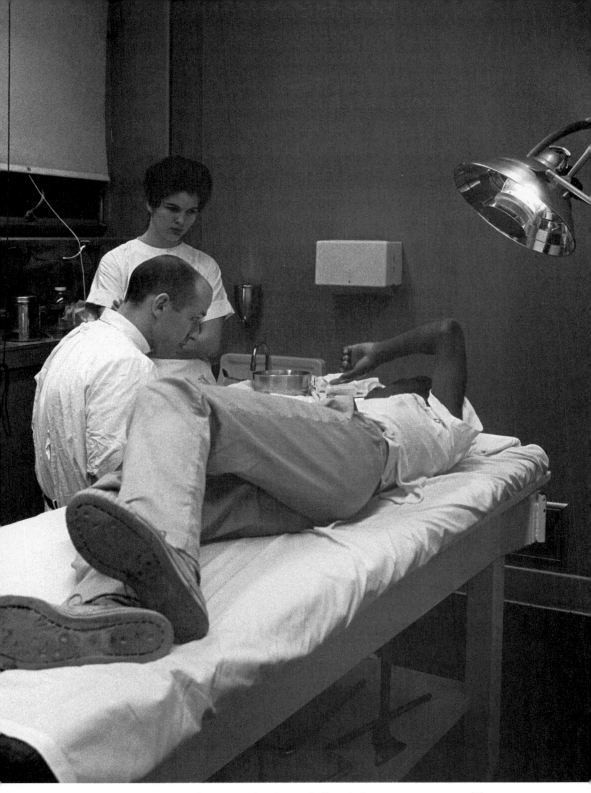

Mixing medications, foods, and illegal drugs can put your life in danger.

THE DRUG ABUSE PREVENTION LIBRARY

DRUG INTERACTIONS:

PROTECTING YOURSELF FROM DANGEROUS DRUG, MEDICATION, AND FOOD COMBINATIONS

Melanie Apel Gordon

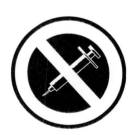

THE ROSEN PUBLISHING GROUP, INC.
NEW YORK

This book is dedicated to my Apel family and my Gordon family for their love, encouragement, support, and belief in me. And, as always, to Amy.

The people pictured in this book are only models. They in no way practice or endorse the activities illustrated. Captions serve only to explain the subjects of photographs and do not in any way imply a connection between the real-life models and the staged situations.

Published in 1999 by The Rosen Publishing Group, Inc.
29 East 21st Street, New York, NY 10010

First Edition

Library of Congress Cataloging-in-Publication Data

Gordon, Melanie Apel.
    Drug interactions : protecting yourself from dangerous drug, medication, and food combinations / Melanie Gordon. -- 1st ed.
        p. cm. -- (The drug abuse prevention library)
    Includes bibliographical references and index.
    Summary: Discusses illegal and legal drugs (both over-the-counter and prescription), alcohol, and food and explains how to prevent dangerous interactions between these substances.
    ISBN 0-8239-2825-X (lib. bdg.)
    1. Drug interactions—United States—Juvenile literature. 2. Drug abuse—United States—Prevention—Juvenile literature. 3. Teenagers—Drug use—United States—Juvenile literature. [1. Drug interactions. 2. Drug abuse.] I. Title. II. Series.
RM302.G67 1999
616'.7045--dc21   98-44974
                                                                  CIP
                                                                   AC

Manufactured in the United States of America

Contents

Introduction

Drugs. Alcohol. You've heard these words. You know what they mean. You probably also know that some drugs are illegal and that it is against the law to drink alcohol if you are under twenty-one years of age. But are you aware that drugs and alcohol by themselves or mixed together can be dangerous, and even deadly? Do you know which drugs, when combined with another drug or with alcohol, can harm or even kill you? When it comes to using drugs and alcohol, what you don't know can hurt you.

Many drugs, especially illegal ones, are harmful to the body. Taking one illegal drug, even alone, is never safe. Mixing it with other drugs, with alcohol, or with certain foods can lead to a dangerous and even fatal interaction.

Being a teenager can be difficult. The stress of growing up causes most young people to wish occasionally that they could escape from their problems. That desire is healthy and normal. For some, however, difficulties seem too tough to handle. These teens may turn to illegal drugs or alcohol, thinking it will help them forget their troubles. That's where the real trouble begins.

Other teens choose not to drink alcohol or use illegal drugs. That doesn't mean that they never take drugs. They may use prescription medications, such as Ritalin, Prozac, or birth-control pills, as ordered by a doctor. They may also take over-the-counter medications, such as aspirin, cold medicine, or diet pills. Although these substances are legal, they still can be harmful if they are not used cautiously and carefully.

As a teenager today, you need to understand the facts about alcohol and drugs—prescription, over-the-counter, and illegal. You need to educate yourself about how all these substances react with one another. When you know the facts, you will be able to make smart choices about using some drugs safely and saying no to other, illegal ones.

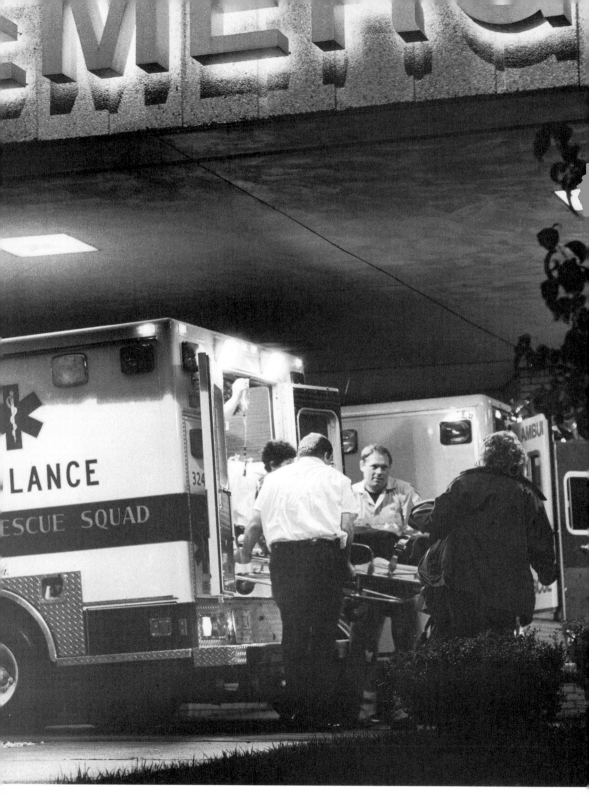
Drugs can interact with one another in dangerous, unpredictable, and even life-threatening ways.

CHAPTER 1

The Basic Facts

"My buddies and I were just having a good time. You know, a little pot, some beer, some coke," says Ty. "But I guess Eric had a little too much.

"When I found Eric lying on the sofa, I couldn't wake him. I called 911. They got him to the hospital just in time. The doctor said that if we had waited any longer, Eric would have died. The doctor also told us that, beside all the stuff Eric did with us, he was taking Zoloft for depression. The combination of alcohol and drugs in his system could have killed him."

Drugs and alcohol—they don't mix. Eric nearly died because of the interaction of alcohol, marijuana, cocaine, and Zoloft in his body.

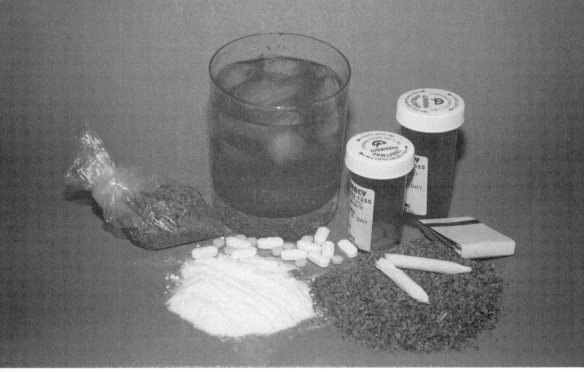

Types of drugs include alcohol, illegal drugs, and prescription and over-the-counter medications.

In order to get the most from this book, you need to be familiar with some terms and ideas about drugs and alcohol. Once you have this information, you will be able to understand how drugs interact and why they can be dangerous. So let's start with the basics.

What Are Drugs and Alcohol?

A drug is a chemical substance that changes the way the body works. Different drugs can affect parts of your body in many ways. Drugs can cause something to happen, prevent something from happening, or stop something that is already happening in your body. The type and amount of a drug and specific instructions (such as

taking it with or without food) can also | *11*
change its effect.

There are three ways you can obtain
drugs.

Over-the-Counter Drugs

Over-the-counter drugs are substances that
you can buy at a store without a prescription. You may be familiar with many over-
the-counter drugs. You've probably used
one or more of them.

Some common over-the-counter medicines or drugs are:

- Acetaminophen (Tylenol), aspirin,
  and ibuprofen, which relieve pain
- Pepto-Bismol, which treats nausea or
  indigestion
- Benadryl, which treats allergies
- Cough drops and throat lozenges,
  which soothe sore throats
- St.-John's-wort, which many people
  use to treat depression

You can probably think of other medicines that you can buy without a prescription at the drugstore, grocery store, or
convenience store.

Most over-the-counter medicines carry a
warning. It advises you to visit your doctor

12 | if the medicine doesn't make you feel better or make your symptoms go away after a short period of time. If you decide you need to see a doctor, he or she will examine you. He or she may then write you a prescription for a stronger or more specialized medicine.

Prescription Drugs

A prescription drug is any drug or medicine that your doctor has to order for you, and that a pharmacist must prepare. Most people at least occasionally need prescription medicines. For example, if you have ever been sick with an infection, pneumonia, or a severe sore throat, your doctor has probably written you a prescription for penicillin or another antibiotic.

However, if you have an illness such as asthma or diabetes, you have to take prescription medicine regularly. Prescription medicines are used not only to treat illnesses; sometimes they are taken for other purposes. For example, many women take prescription birth-control pills to prevent pregnancy.

As you learned earlier, you may need to take prescription medication if over-the-counter medicine is not powerful enough to take care of your problem. For example,

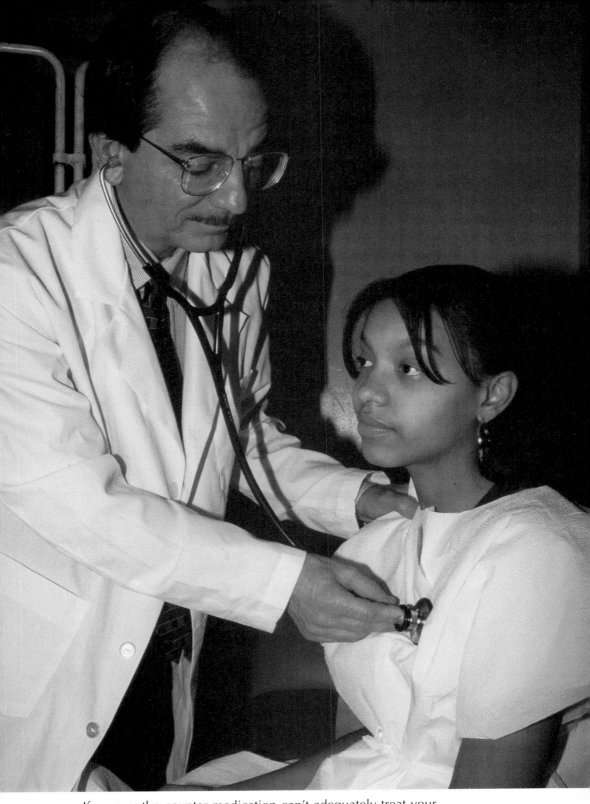

If an over-the-counter medication can't adequately treat your condition, your doctor may prescribe a prescription drug.

14 if you have broken your arm, an over-the-counter drug, such as acetaminophen, would probably not be able to take away all your pain. Your doctor would likely write a prescription for a stronger painkiller, such as Vicodin. Or if you suffer from severe migraine headaches, you need more than aspirin to get rid of them. You probably need a prescription medication.

If you finish all of the medicine your doctor has prescribed but still don't feel better, you will have to visit your doctor again. Your doctor may prescribe more of the same medicine, a different medicine, or no medicine at all. Prescription drugs can be very dangerous, and doctors are careful how much they prescribe and for whom.

Illegal Drugs

Illegal drugs are substances you buy from drug dealers, or from someone who is not legally licensed to sell drugs. Illegal drugs are extremely dangerous. You rarely know or can trust the person who is selling them. You also don't know what other substances have been mixed with the drug. Often drug dealers mix an illegal drug with another substance so that they have more product to sell.

For example, a dealer might mix cocaine

with talcum powder, sugar, or another, cheaper drug. If you use illegal drugs, you simply cannot be sure what substances you are putting into your body.

Illegal drugs are usually used recreationally, or for fun, not because the person using them has an illness or injury. They can be very addictive. People often like the way they feel on illegal drugs. And they usually don't like the way they feel when the drug wears off. So they take more of an illegal drug to feel good again.

You may be asking yourself, Couldn't this also happen with a prescription drug, such as a painkiller? The answer is yes. People can become addicted to prescription drugs. But, remember, prescription drug use is carefully monitored by a doctor. Your doctor will help ensure that you don't take too much of a prescription drug, take it for too long, or take it for the wrong reasons. However, if you are using illegal drugs, there is no one to give you guidance and to help ensure that you don't overdose (take too much) or become addicted.

Why Use or Abuse?

Why do teens use illegal drugs and alcohol? The teenage years are filled with change, confusion, and turmoil. Some teens may

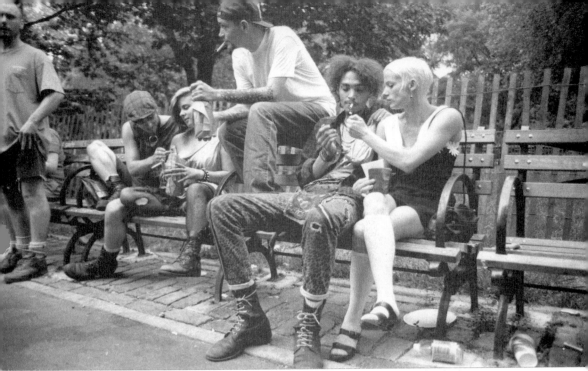

Teens use illegal drugs for many reasons. Some think drugs are cool or fun, and others use them to cope with problems.

find it difficult to cope with life at home or at school. Family problems, such as illness, abuse, alcoholism, or divorce, may be hard to handle. Poor grades, behavioral problems, or the desire to be popular may make school stressful and painful. Teens may turn to illegal drugs or alcohol because they think doing so will numb their pain and make life more bearable.

Other teens think it's fun or cool to use illegal drugs or alcohol. They may feel as though they have to use them to be popular and accepted by their friends. Peer pressure—when people your age try to persuade you to do something you don't want to do—can be very powerful and very hard to resist.

The truth is this: Using illegal drugs or alcohol can never solve your problems; it can only add to them. Alcohol is a drug. It's illegal to drink alcohol if you are under twenty-one years of age, and it's illegal to use certain drugs no matter how old you are. If you're caught using, carrying, or selling, you can be arrested, fined, and put in jail.

More important, illegal drugs and alcohol can mess you up. They can damage your brain, make you sick, and even keep you from being able to have children. Illegal drugs and alcohol can make you do foolish and risky things. They can kill you.

"My best friend, Mia, had just moved away, and then I found out that my parents were getting divorced," says Alexis.

"I felt so alone. I had no one to talk to about how it felt to lose all of these important people at the same time. So I started drinking a lot. I knew some guys at school who smoked pot, and I started hanging out with them. I thought that if I drank and smoked pot, I wouldn't have to think about my problems. I thought they would just go away. But I was wrong."

Common Types of Illegal Drugs
Most teens have heard of marijuana and cocaine. These are two of the most commonly

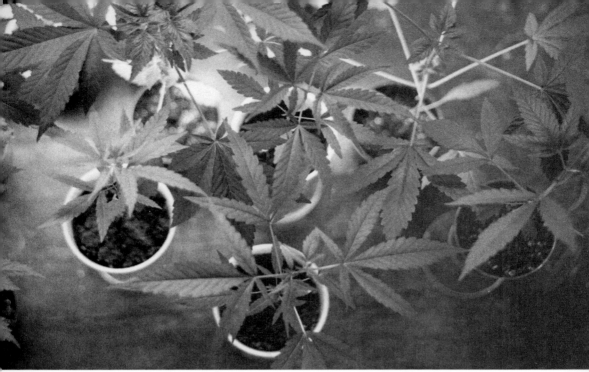

Marijuana, often known as pot, is a popular illegal drug among teens.

used illegal, or street, drugs. But there are many others. You may recognize some of them by their street names.

Marijuana

Marijuana, commonly known as pot, is the most widely used illegal drug in the United States. It tends to be the first illegal drug used by teens. Marijuana blocks messages going to your brain and changes the way your mind sees things. Your emotions, vision, hearing, and coordination can all suffer if you are using marijuana.

Short-term effects of marijuana use range from sleepiness to memory problems, bloodshot eyes, and dry mouth. Long-term effects include an increased risk of cancer, infertility (being unable to have children), and low sex drive.

Cocaine
Cocaine is a stimulant, a drug that speeds up your bodily processes. Its street name is coke. Crack cocaine is a smokable form of cocaine. It makes you feel as if you have limitless power or energy. However, when cocaine wears off, it leaves you depressed, edgy, and craving more. Cocaine's effects include increased blood pressure, heart rate, breathing rate, and body temperature. It also causes confusion, violent behavior, and heart attacks.

Methamphetamine
Methamphetamine is another stimulant. It affects the central nervous system (CNS). Its street names include speed, meth, and crank. If you use methamphetamine, you may feel your heart beating faster, have feelings of euphoria (extreme happiness), or experience insomnia (inability to sleep). You may also lose weight, have a fever, and feel irritable, confused, anxious, or paranoid.

Hallucinogens
Hallucinogens are drugs that confuse the way people see reality. Names, or nicknames, for some hallucinogens are acid, PCP, angel dust, LSD, and magic mushrooms.

20 Under the influence of these drugs, you lose your senses of direction, distance, and time. They may also cause unpredictable, erratic, and violent behavior.

Inhalants

Inhalants are drugs that are sniffed to cause a high. They include a variety of chemicals found in aerosol sprays, cleaning products, and glue. Inhalants are easy to get, but they are extremely harmful. Inhaling chemicals may cause numbness, headaches, muscle weakness, and stomach pain. It may also lead to suffocation, hallucinations, brain damage, and sudden death.

Narcotics

Narcotics are pain relievers. Common narcotics are codeine, heroin, methadone, and morphine. Doctors sometimes prescribe narcotics, and, if used as your doctor instructs, they are safe. Narcotics become unsafe when you use more than the doctor directs or when you get them from a dealer on the street. Narcotics make you feel relaxed, sleepy, and very happy. They take away pain, but only briefly. Once the pain returns, you need more of these drugs.

Some people become addicted to narcotics because they like the way narcotics make them feel. But narcotics may cause

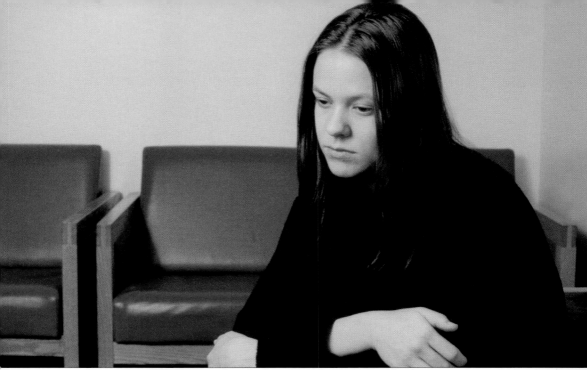

Illegal drugs can cause depression, mood swings, and other serious physical and psychological problems.

serious problems. Some problems you may experience include mood swings, shaking, and constipation. They may even stop your breathing. People who inject narcotics, such as heroin, and share needles are at risk for HIV, the virus that causes AIDS.

Now You Know

Now you've learned the basic facts about prescription, over-the-counter, and illegal drugs. You know what they are and, for illegal drugs, what they do. Seems simple, right? It's not that easy. Drugs are often unpredictable, especially when used in combination with other drugs, food, or alcohol. The next chapter explains some ways drugs interact with one another.

CHAPTER 2

Defining a Drug Interaction

A drug interaction occurs when two or more substances are taken together and their combination causes a reaction in the body. These two substances can be a drug and alcohol, two different drugs, or a drug and a certain food. There are three types of drug interactions.

Additive Interactions

Additive interactions happen when one drug adds to the effect of another drug. For example, if you are taking certain prescription drugs for a migraine headache, and then drink alcohol, you will feel confused and disoriented. This effect occurs because the medicine and alcohol combine to slow down your body and brain more than just one substance would have if used alone.

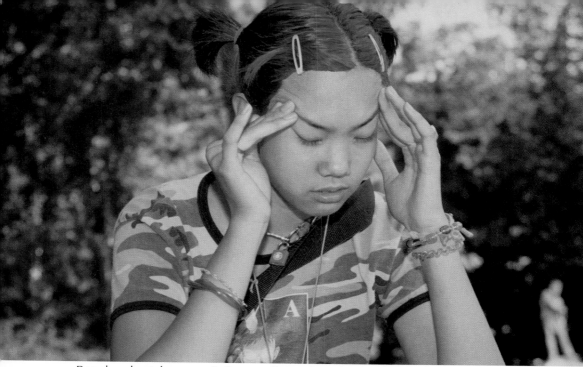

People who take prescription medicine for migraine headaches can't drink alcohol, because the two drugs will interact.

Antagonistic Interactions

Antagonistic interactions happen when one drug cancels out the effects of another drug. If a woman taking birth-control pills needs to take an antibiotic, she must use another form of birth control while using the antibiotic. The antibiotic may cause the birth-control pill to fail. Antagonistic interactions can be especially dangerous when one of the drugs is needed to keep a person healthy or alive, such as an antiseizure drug for epilepsy or an antirejection drug for transplanted organs.

Unpredictable Interactions

Unpredictable interactions occur when two substances react in an unexpected way.

24 These are the scariest type of interactions, because one usually cannot predict them. They also take the longest to be noticed. For example, a person may take a drug for an allergy. Over time, this medicine builds up in his or her body. Then, when he or she takes another drug for a different problem, the two drugs interact in ways no one expects. Combining two substances can cause symptoms as mild as a rash and dizziness or as severe as a heart attack.

All of these interactions can happen to people using prescription drugs, over-the-counter drugs, illegal drugs, or alcohol. That's why knowing about drug interactions is so important.

"A whole bunch of us were doing drugs one night," says Sam. "I don't even remember all the stuff we were taking. We were drinking, using pot and cocaine, and taking some prescription painkiller that one of the guys had stolen from his mother's medicine cabinet. We were mixing it all together, but I didn't think that would matter.

"We decided to go for a walk. Danielle climbed up onto the railing of a bridge. She must have been hallucinating because she thought she was on a tightrope. She yelled,

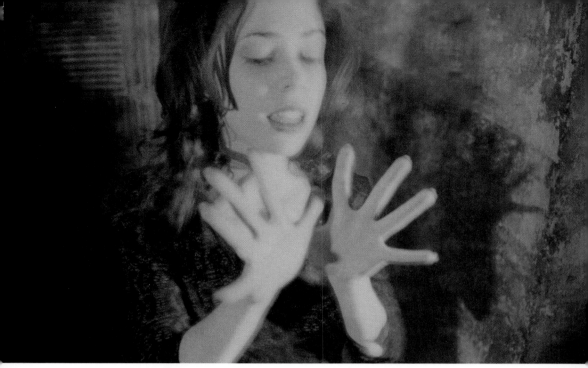

Unpredictable interactions can be terrifying because they are unexpected and often hard to identify.

'Look at me! I'm a tightrope walker!' She tried to balance on one foot.

"Danielle lost her balance on the bridge railing and fell off. I haven't touched drugs or alcohol since that night. Seeing her dead body on the ground below was the worst experience of my life. I still have nightmares about it."

Illegal Drugs Don't Mix

Danielle mixed several types of illegal drugs with alcohol and a prescription drug. It's very difficult to predict how a combination of drugs will affect your body and mind. In her case, by the time anyone knew, it was too late.

25

26   Most illegal drugs interact with each other in one of two ways:

- The interaction slows down all your body's systems, including your breathing rate, heart rate, and blood pressure. You become extremely relaxed but unable to think clearly. Because your breathing and heart slow down, you can become unconscious or even die.
- The interaction speeds up all your body's systems, including your breathing rate, heart rate, and blood pressure. It makes you feel as if you are bigger than life. You feel as if you can do anything and as if nothing can hurt you. This interaction puts you at risk for dangerous behavior that you wouldn't consider under normal circumstances.

You have no way of knowing how drugs will interact in your body. If you use prescription or over-the-counter medication, ask your doctor or a pharmacist what precautions to take. When it comes to illegal drugs, the best way to stay safe is to say no.

CHAPTER 3

What About Alcohol?

*A*lcohol is found in drinks such as beer, wine, and liquors. Alcohol is a drug. It is a depressant, which means it slows the body's systems. It can make a person feel relaxed, powerful, brave, silly, or sexy. When you drink too much alcohol, your body can't get rid of it quickly enough. It poisons your blood, making you drunk. You become clumsy, your speech slurs, and it becomes difficult to walk and balance. If you continue drinking alcohol, your body may start to shut down. You may pass out, fall into a coma, and even die.

Alcohol and Its Effects
Drinking alcohol depresses your central nervous system. The following list explains how alcohol can affect you.

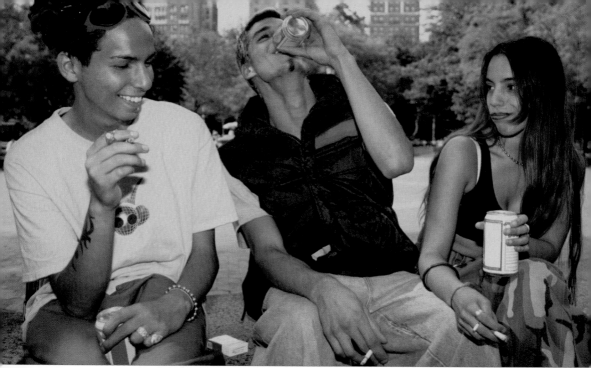

At first alcohol may make you feel lighthearted and giddy, but later you may become emotional and depressed.

- Vision: It may be blurry or doubled.
- Perceptions: The world may appear different from actuality.
- Emotions: You may initially become happy and silly but then later become upset and overly emotional.
- Judgment: It will be impaired, or weakened. For example, you may think you can safely drive a car, but you won't be able to judge the amount of time you need to stop or how close you are to objects on the roadside.

If you use alcohol over a long period of time, you can seriously damage your liver. Liver damage can cause all kinds of physical problems, including cirrhosis, a fatal disease. A damaged liver also speeds up the rate at which some drugs are metabolized, or used by the body. Certain prescription drugs that people may need to stay alive do not work well if they don't stay in the body long enough to do their jobs. As you can see, alcohol abuse can severely harm your health.

Defining Alcoholism

Alcoholism is a disease, just as drug addiction is. A person who is called an alcoholic is addicted to alcohol. An alcoholic is physically and psychologically dependent upon the drug. Without it, he or she cannot function well in daily life.

Alcoholics usually begin as social drinkers, drinking alcohol occasionally at parties and special events. However, alcoholics lose control of their drinking. They may drink larger quantities of alcohol and do so more often. Eventually, alcohol becomes the most important thing in their lives, even more important than school, a job, family, or friends.

Some alcoholics drink to escape problems, but alcohol can only increase their problems. If you or someone you know shows signs of being an alcoholic, help is

30 available. Check the section called Where to Go for Help at the end of this book, or look in your local phone book for hotlines, information, and support groups for alcoholics.

Alcoholics are at special risk for drug interactions. Since they often have alcohol in their bodies, it can be difficult for them to use over-the-counter or prescription medication safely. Also, because of the alcohol present, these drugs may not affect the body in the way that they should. Finally, until alcoholics are able to stop drinking, they cannot use any medication that will interact negatively with alcohol. If they need this medication to get well or to live, being unable to take it can have severe consequences.

Mixing Alcohol with Legal Drugs

Many legal drugs, whether they are prescription or over-the-counter, can also become very dangerous when combined with alcohol. Because so many types of drugs exist, it's impossible to discuss all of them. Here are some examples of the most common alcohol and drug interactions.

Alcohol and antihistamines, when mixed, disturb psychomotor performance, which is the way your body reacts to what your brain tells it to do. Antihistamines are

drugs many people take to relieve their
allergy symptoms. Antihistamines usually come with a warning label telling you not to drive or work with heavy machinery because the drug may make you feel drowsy and less alert. The warning also tells you to avoid drinking alcohol while you are taking the antihistamine because it will increase these effects.

Alcohol and some antibiotics taken together may give you a headache and an upset stomach. Antibiotics are prescription medicines taken to fight infections. Alcohol can also stop certain antibiotics from working in your body.

Alcohol and aspirin, when taken together, prolong the time that it takes for your blood to clot, or clump. When your blood clots, your body stops bleeding. Because they slow clotting, aspirin and alcohol increase bleeding time. For example, if you are using aspirin as a painkiller after surgery, the aspirin makes the bleeding you experience last longer. If you then drink alcohol while you are taking aspirin, it will take even longer for bleeding to stop.

Alcohol and sleeping pills can really knock you out. You will feel drowsy and uncoordinated. Your reaction time will slow. Some sleeping pills are long-lasting,

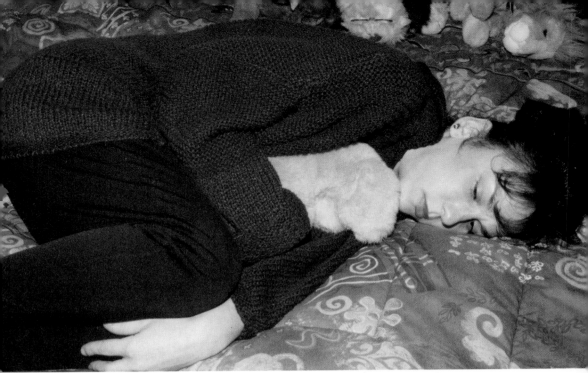

You should never mix sleeping pills with alcohol. They can interact to cause coma or even death.

which means that the effects last longer than a normal dose. Even if you take these pills at night, if you drink alcohol as late as the next afternoon, you will have problems with your coordination and concentration. If you take too many sleeping pills or take them with alcohol, you may fall into a sleep so deep that it will be very difficult, if not impossible, to wake up. If you cannot wake up, you can slip into a coma and die.

Mixing Alcohol with Illegal Drugs

The effects of alcohol or illegal drugs, even when taken separately, can be very dangerous. When the two are mixed together, they can be deadly.

With Barbiturates

If you drink alcohol and take another depressant drug, such as a barbiturate, an additive interaction occurs. Barbiturates include many tranquilizers, sleeping pills, and sedatives. The interaction causes your body to slow down even more than it would using alcohol alone.

The alcohol and the drug multiply each other's effects on your body. These two depressants act together to strongly depress your CNS, or central nervous system. Your breathing and heart drastically slow down and could even stop. Your alertness, concentration, coordination, and judgment are also impaired. Adding alcohol to barbiturates, whether you are using them as prescription or recreational drugs, could cost you your life. Comedians John Belushi and Chris Farley both died as a result of combining alcohol with barbiturates.

With Narcotics

If you're using narcotics, such as morphine or heroin, drinking alcohol will strengthen the effects of these drugs. Like barbiturates, narcotics depress your CNS. You will feel your breathing and heart rate slow down. They could actually slow so much that they eventually stop. Again, you could die.

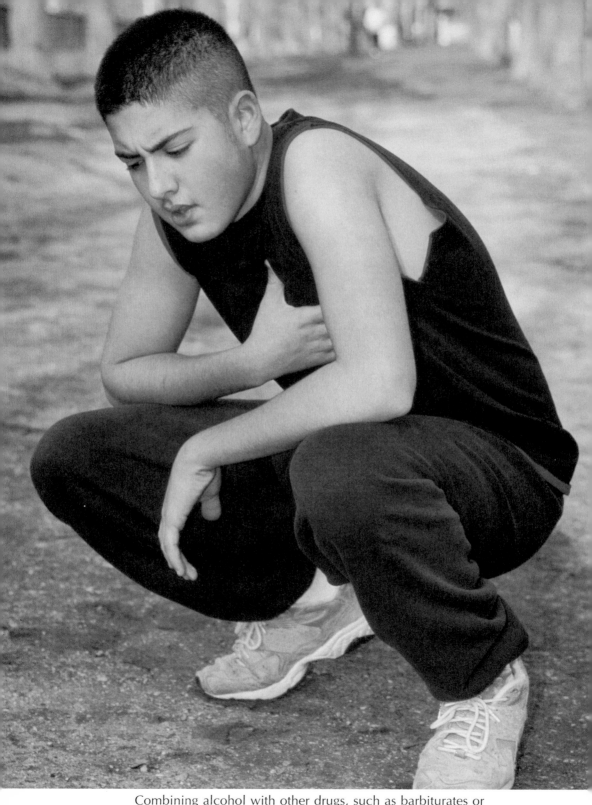
Combining alcohol with other drugs, such as barbiturates or narcotics, can affect your heart and breathing rates.

With Marijuana

The combination of alcohol and marijuana causes a decrease in alertness, as well as a decrease in motor and intellectual skills. This means that your actions and thoughts are slower than normal. Activities such as driving a car, having a conversation, writing a paper for school, or performing daily tasks become difficult.

Ordinary, everyday things may seem silly, funny, or more important than usual. For example, a situation that you might normally consider quite serious may seem very entertaining, and you may not be able to stop laughing. Or something that would not normally bother you may become extremely upsetting.

With Stimulants

Alcohol and stimulant drugs, such as cocaine and methamphetamine, may perk you up and make you feel more energetic. However, this feeling lasts only a little while. When the good feelings wear off, you become tired and depressed. This low feeling usually makes the user want more stimulant and alcohol. The user may take more of the drug and alcohol, but eventually he or she once again feels exhausted and depressed.

36 Can you see where this is going? Can you see the vicious cycle? This cycle of highs and lows often leads to addiction. People can become addicted to all types of drugs. As time goes by, the user builds up a tolerance to the drug and alcohol. This means that the person needs larger amounts to feel the way he or she once did after using smaller amounts. Once someone has become addicted to a drug, it is extremely difficult to stop using it.

Addiction is very scary. It destroys lives and relationships with family and friends. Also, many drug users die from overdoses, since they need to keep increasing their drug intake. Luckily, there are drug abuse centers, hotlines, and support groups for people who want to end their addiction to drugs or alcohol.

To protect yourself from drug interactions, read the warning labels attached to all prescription and over-the-counter medications. Always ask your doctor or pharmacist if your medication will interact with alcohol. Since illegal drugs do not come with warning labels or product information, you should never take them. Be smart and assume that you will suffer consequences if you mix any drug with alcohol.

CHAPTER 4

Mixing Drugs with Food

"I was taking an anti-inflammatory medicine for an injury I got playing football," says Calvin, *"but I didn't read the label on the bottle of pills very carefully. The warning said not to take the drug with food, especially salty food. I ate a bag of potato chips right after I took the pills. Boy, did I have a stomachache! I was in worse pain from my stomach than I was from the injury."*

What About Food?

A drug-food interaction occurs when a food you eat affects a drug you are taking. Because of the substances in food, the medicine does not work the way it should. It may work faster, slower, or not at all.

Food does not affect all drugs, but it can

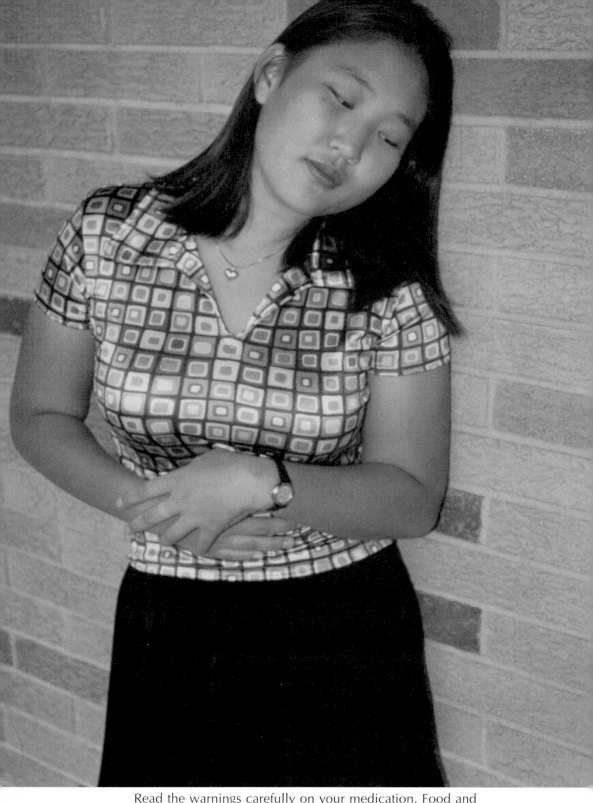

Read the warnings carefully on your medication. Food and drugs can interact to produce painful side effects.

interact with many of them. Certain foods |
may slow the action of some drugs. If you
have food in your stomach, other drugs
won't be absorbed (soaked up) well in your
body. If your body cannot absorb the
drugs, then the drugs will not work. You
must take these drugs one hour before you
eat or two hours afterward. Other medicines cause stomach discomfort if you
don't take them with food. You must take
these immediately after you eat a meal.

Here are some common food-drug
interactions:

- The calcium in dairy products, such
  as milk, cheese, and ice cream,
  makes it difficult for the body to
  absorb some antibiotics. One of
  these is tetracycline, an antibiotic
  often used for acne.
- Soft drinks and fruit and vegetable
  juices with high amounts of acid, such
  as apple, grape, orange, and tomato,
  cause some drugs to dissolve in the
  stomach instead of in the intestines,
  where they are better absorbed.
- Foods that contain a substance
  called tyramine react very badly
  with drugs prescribed for severe

40

depression, called MAO inhibitors, and drugs prescribed for high blood pressure. These foods—cheese, sausages, yogurt, sour cream, bananas, and avocados, to name a few—can cause blood pressure to rise to dangerous levels when mixed with these drugs. These combinations can even be fatal.

A Checklist

Ask your doctor if the drug you are taking should be taken with or without food. Also ask him or her if you should avoid certain foods while taking the drug. You should always:

- Read the label. If you don't understand something or need more information, ask your doctor or your pharmacist.
- Read the directions, warnings, and interaction precautions on prescription and over-the-counter drugs.
- Take medicines with a full glass of water.
- Unless your doctor tells you to do so, don't stir medicines into food or take capsules apart. This can affect the way the drug is absorbed into your system.

- Vitamins and minerals can interact with some drugs. Don't take them at the same time as your medication.
- Don't mix medicines with hot drinks. The heat may destroy the drugs' effectiveness.

If you think that you are experiencing a drug-food interaction, tell someone immediately. If the interaction seems minor, call your doctor or pharmacist. Do this right away, because you cannot predict whether the effects will worsen. If the effects are more serious, call 911. Acting quickly can prevent serious consequences or even save your life.

CHAPTER 5

Using Prescription Drugs Safely

"*I take theophylline to control my asthma,*" *says Miranda. "I was having trouble sleeping last year, so a friend gave me some barbiturates to help. They didn't help me sleep. In fact, they made my body get rid of the theophylline too fast, and I had a really bad asthma attack. I ended up in the hospital, where it's really hard to get any sleep!*"

Miranda mixed a prescription medicine with an illegally obtained prescription drug. The combination could have killed her. Miranda should have told her doctor that she was having trouble sleeping. Her doctor could have prescribed a drug for her that would not have interacted with her asthma medication.

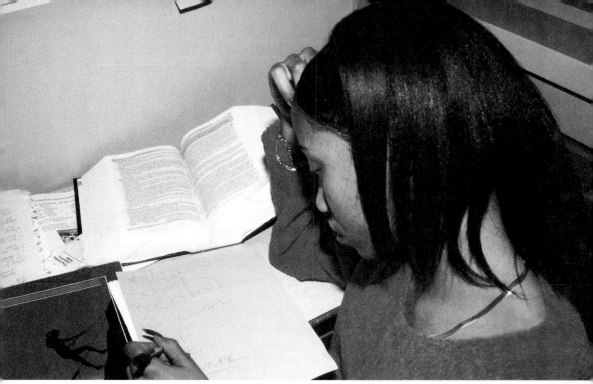
Many teens with attention deficit disorder (ADD) take the pre-scription drug Ritalin to help them concentrate.

Why Have a Prescription?

There are many reasons your doctor might prescribe medicine for you. You may have had a prescription medicine for a cold, cough, allergy, menstrual cramps, migraine headaches, or asthma. Or you may have had one for diarrhea, birth control, attention deficit disorder (ADD), irritable bowel syndrome, pain from broken bones, or lots of other things.

Some people with ADD, or a similar disorder called ADHD, take a prescription drug called Ritalin. Those suffering from depression may use Prozac or Zoloft. Other medicines that may sound familiar to you are Claritin for allergies, Vicodin and codeine

43

44 | to kill pain, and naproxen for menstrual cramps. If you have asthma, you may be taking Azmacort, Beclovent, Proventil, Alupent, Intal, or AeroBid. Antibiotics such as penicillin, Keflex, erythromycin, Bactrim, Cipro, tetracycline, and Flagyl can treat strep throat, pneumonia, bad acne, or a fungal infection. These are just a few of the most popular prescription drugs. There are many, many more.

Prescription Drugs and Illegal Drugs

Since prescription drugs can treat so many problems, it's likely that you are using one now or have been recently. It may be hard for you to find information on interactions between prescription and illegal drugs. The best thing to do is ask your doctor.

Most likely, the combination will be harmful. If illegal drugs or alcohol cause the prescription drug not to work as well as it should, you will remain ill. If it causes an unexpected reaction, such as vomiting, convulsions, or unconsciousness, you could die.

Prescription Drugs and Legal Drugs

The fact that some drugs are legal does not mean that they're risk-free. Did you know that some cough medicines contain alcohol? If you take cough medicine, be sure to

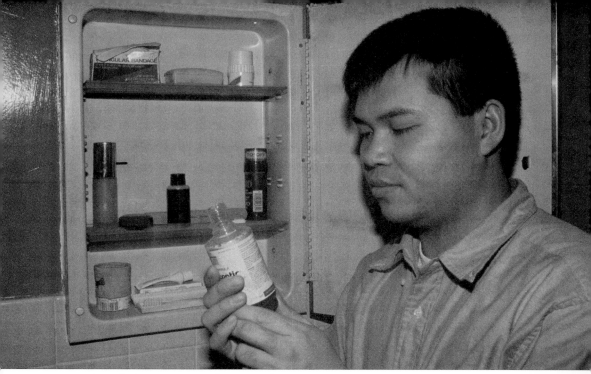

Simply because you don't need a prescription to purchase over-the-counter drugs doesn't mean that they are always safe.

choose one that is alcohol-free. The others could react badly with certain drugs.

Or did you know that erythromycin, an antibiotic, can prevent your body from getting rid of caffeine? Caffeine is a drug found in coffee, chocolate, and some soft drinks. As it builds up in your body, caffeine can cause tremors, or shaking, and high blood pressure.

To understand the way in which prescription drugs can interact with other prescription and over-the-counter drugs, let's look at an example.

Tetracycline is a popular antibiotic used to treat severe acne. This prescription drug should not be taken with antacids. Antacids, which soothe ulcers, cause tetracycline to be

45

46 less effective. Someone using tetracycline should avoid iron and zinc supplements, which have the same effect. That person should also avoid Pepto-Bismol, an over-the-counter medicine taken for an upset stomach. Pepto-Bismol causes tetracycline to be poorly absorbed in your body, making it less effective. As you can see, one drug can react in many ways with many types of drugs.

These are just some interactions that can occur between prescription drugs and other prescription or over-the-counter drugs. Avoid mixing any one medication with another without first talking with your doctor. Be sure your doctor knows about every drug you take. The best way to stay healthy is to keep both yourself and your doctor informed.

Drug and Alcohol Sense

"*My* *school is doing a drug and alcohol awareness program this year,*" *says Jared.* "*We learn about alcohol and drugs and how they affect people. We also talk about drug interactions and drug safety.*

"*At first I figured all this would be a waste of time, but it's actually been pretty useful. I've been sick a few times this year, and it was helpful to know what I could and couldn't take with my medicines. I also found out that I couldn't drink alcohol while I was taking them, which I didn't know before.*"

Jared's school is conducting a very useful and important program. It's teaching him that he is responsible for himself and for the drugs he puts into his body. Jared has

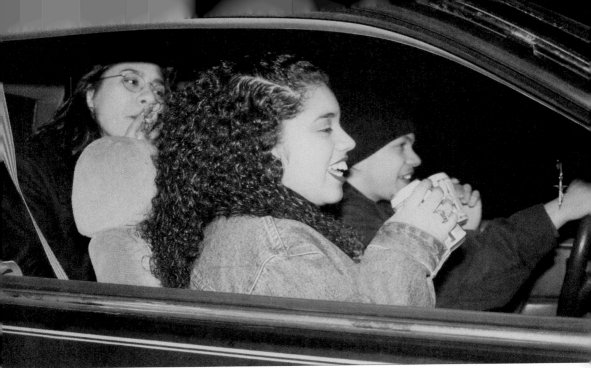

Drunk drivers kill thousands of innocent people each year.

already learned tips about alcohol and other drugs that are helping him stay safe and healthy.

Making Smart Decisions About Alcohol

You already know that alcohol is a drug and that it doesn't mix with other drugs. But there are other safety precautions that you need to take when drinking alcohol.

Drinking and Driving

If you have been drinking, driving a car not only puts you at risk, it also risks the lives of other passengers, drivers, and pedestrians. If you are not willing to refrain from drinking, appoint a designated driver. A designated driver is a person who agrees to stay sober all evening so that he or she can drive everyone else home safely. If no one is sober at the evening's end, consider staying overnight, calling a cab, or even calling your parents. Of course, your parents will not be happy that you are drunk, but they will realize that you are being responsible by asking to be picked up and driven home.

Water Safety

Drinking alcohol at the beach, near a pool, or on a boat may seem like fun. But beware! You may find yourself in a very dangerous situation. When you drink too much alcohol, your judgment becomes impaired. You may be willing to take risks that you wouldn't normally consider. When drunk, you may decide to go for a swim. You may get lost in the water or even forget how to swim. Can you see why so many drownings are linked to alcohol?

Sexual Choices

Sex and alcohol are another bad combination. Many teens regret getting drunk and having sex recklessly or impulsively. Because they were drunk, they weren't thinking clearly. Other teenagers get drunk and forget to use protection. Unprotected

50 | sex can lead to pregnancy and to HIV and AIDS and other sexually transmitted diseases. Mixing alcohol with sex can destroy your reputation, health, and future.

It's best to avoid drinking alcohol until you are old enough to drink legally and responsibly. However, if you are going to drink alcohol, you may want to set limits ahead of time. Before you start drinking, decide when and where you will or won't drink alcohol. Decide how much you'll drink and when you'll stop. Decide what you will or will not do while you are drinking. And stand by your decisions, no matter what anyone else says or how you feel when drinking. You may want to share your decisions with a close friend. That way, if things start to get out of control, he or she can remind you about the promises you made to yourself.

What About Smoking?

Just a few words about drugs and cigarettes. Cigarettes speed up your body's metabolism of certain drugs so the drugs don't stay in the body long enough to complete their jobs. These drugs include theophylline (an asthma drug), pentazocine (a painkiller), and some tranquilizers, analgesics (painkillers), and antidepressants. If

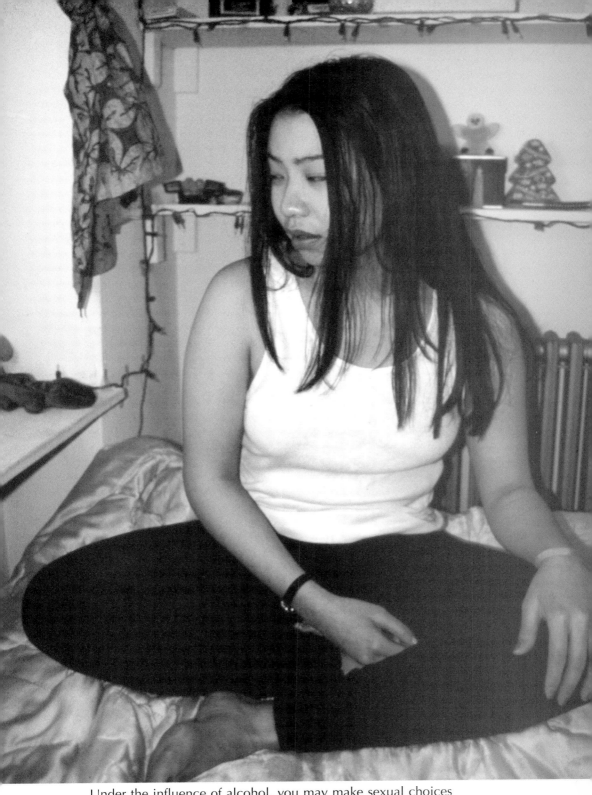
Under the influence of alcohol, you may make sexual choices
that you later regret.

52 you are a smoker and need any of these medications, you will have to take larger doses than normal. If you stop smoking, the dosage will have to be changed so that you get a smaller, more appropriate amount of the drug.

For this reason, it's very important that your doctor knows whether or not you smoke. If he or she isn't aware that you're a smoker, he or she may not prescribe enough medicine. If you quit smoking but forget to tell your doctor this, your prescription will be stronger than necessary. You will risk an accidental overdose.

In addition, girls who smoke cigarettes and take birth-control pills increase their risk of having a heart attack, breast cancer, or a stroke. Yes, these things really can happen to young people, even teens!

Safety and Illegal Drugs

There is nothing safe about illegal drugs. The smartest way to avoid problems with them is to avoid the drugs themselves. However, if you are using illegal drugs, there are a few things you can do to protect yourself.

- Don't drink alcohol when you are using drugs.

- Don't mix drugs. Take only one at a time and don't take another drug until the effects of the first drug have worn off.
- Do not share needles with other drug users. Sharing needles can result in the spread of HIV and AIDS.
- Know your drug dealer. A dealer you do not know well may try to slip another substance into a drug.

Drug abuse often leads to addiction. If you are currently using illegal drugs, you can get help. You can talk to a parent, close friend, relative, teacher, or guidance counselor. There are also many organizations that treat and counsel teens who use illegal drugs. Where to Go for Help at the back of this book lists some phone numbers you can call to get information and assistance.

"Two years ago, I started seeing a psychiatrist. I was depressed all the time. She gave me a prescription for Prozac, an antidepressant. It really helped, and I was much happier for a while. Then everything changed.

"The following spring, I went to another doctor because my allergies had gotten pretty bad. He put me on an antihistamine called

54 *Periactin. I didn't tell him about the Prozac because it didn't seem important.*

"All of a sudden, my depression came back. I went to my psychiatrist, and she started asking me about my health, so I mentioned the Periactin. She explained that Periactin and Prozac caused something called an antagonistic interaction. Basically, the allergy drug kept the antidepressant from working. To get rid of my depression, she said that one of the drugs would have to be changed to a different drug."

Prescription Smarts

Sometimes people experience drug interactions because their doctors do not know about all the drugs they are taking. You should give your doctor a list of all the drugs you take, including illegal ones. Be honest. If you are on birth-control pills, smoking cigarettes, or doing something illegal, it's important for your doctor to know. This will make it easier for him or her to prescribe medicine to take care of your illness.

If you have questions about possible side effects or interactions, ask your doctor. Also, be sure you understand exactly how to take the medication. It is so important to take the medicines exactly the way your doctor directs. Often, when your pharmacist

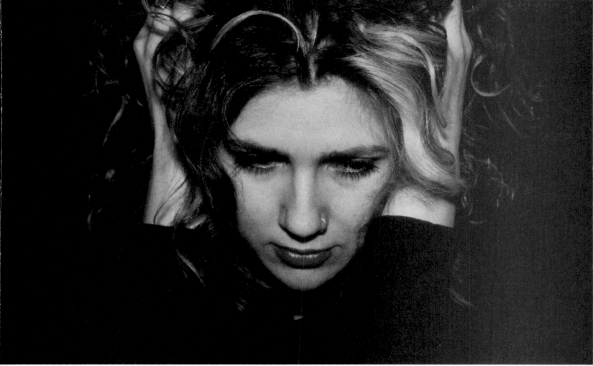

If you experience side effects, such as depression, from your medication, contact your doctor or pharmacist immediately.

fills your prescription, he or she will give you a list of things, such as other drugs, foods, or alcohol, that won't mix well with your prescription. You should read this list very carefully.

If you're taking an over-the-counter medication, read the label and follow the directions. If you have questions, ask your pharmacist.

Sharing Information with Your Doctor

Whenever you are given a prescription for a drug, ask your doctor:

- The name of the medicine
- What it's supposed to do
- What side effects might occur

56

- How long you should take the medicine (Always take the medicine for as long as you're supposed to. Don't stop taking it because you feel better.)
- If there are any drugs you should not take while you are taking this one
- If there are any foods or beverages you should avoid
- If you can drink alcohol with the medicine
- If the prescription can be refilled without an appointment, or if you need to visit the doctor again

Tell your doctor if you:

- Have allergic reactions, such as headaches or rashes, to drugs or foods
- Are taking any other medicines, such as birth-control pills or insulin, or any illegal or over-the-counter drugs
- Use alcohol or tobacco
- Are on a special diet or are taking vitamins or minerals
- Are being treated for another condition by another doctor
- Are pregnant or breast-feeding
- Have diabetes or kidney or liver disease
- Feel that the prescription drug isn't doing what it's supposed to do

- Have an unexpected reaction (report this immediately)

One last thing to remember: Do not share prescription medicine with anyone. Only the person whose name is on the prescription should take the medicine. If a person takes a prescription drug meant for someone other than himself or herself, a harmful interaction can occur.

So now you know the facts. You are educated about drugs and their effects. You understand what can happen if you mix one drug with another or with alcohol. And, most important, you know that your body belongs to you and no one else. When it comes to drugs, choose wisely to protect your health, your safety, and your future.

Glossary

additive interaction When one substance increases the effect of another substance.

alcoholism Addiction to alcohol.

antagonistic interaction When one substance cancels out the effect of another substance.

antibiotic Prescription medicine taken to fight infection.

antihistamine Medicine taken to relieve cold and allergy symptoms.

barbiturates Type of depressant drug, such as sleeping pills or tranquilizers.

delusion Strongly held but false and often bizarre belief.

depressant Drug that slows down the body and mind.

drug Chemical substance that changes the way the body works.

hallucination Perception of an object
that does not actually exist.

hallucinogen Drug that confuses the
way people experience reality.

illegal drug Drug that is outlawed, or a
prescription drug bought from
someone not legally licensed to sell it.

inhalant Chemical that is sniffed to get
high.

interact To act upon one another.

interaction When two or more substances act upon one another.

methamphetamine Stimulant drug
that affects the central nervous system.

narcotic Illegal or prescription drug
used to relieve pain.

over-the-counter drug Drug that can
be purchased without a prescription.

paranoia State of feeling suspicious,
anxious, and uneasy.

prescription drug Drug that must be
ordered by a doctor and prepared by a
pharmacist.

stimulant Drug that speeds up the
body and mind.

unpredictable interaction When one
drug, taken over a period of time,
builds up and reacts with another
drug.

Where to Go for Help

Alcoholics Anonymous (AA)
P.O. Box 459
Grand Central Station
New York, NY 10163
(212) 870-3400
Web site: http://www.alcoholics-anonymous.org

American Pharmaceutical Association (APhA)
2215 Constitution Avenue NW
Washington, DC 20037
(202) 628-4410
Web site: http://www.aphanet.org

Center for Substance Abuse Prevention (CSAP)
5600 Fishers Lane
Rockwall II Building, Suite 900
Rockville, MD 20857
(301) 443-0365
Web site: http://www.samhsa.gov
e-mail: nnadal@samhsa.gov

Narcotics Anonymous (NA)
World Service Office
P.O. Box 9999

Van Nuys, CA 91409

(818) 773-9999

Web site: http://www.wsoinc.com

e-mail: wso@aol.com

National Clearinghouse for Alcohol and Drug Information (NCADI)

P.O. Box 2345

Rockville, MD 20847

(800) 729-6686

(301) 468-2600

Web site: http://www.health.org

e-mail: info@prevline.health.org

United States Food and Drug Administration (FDA)

5600 Fishers Lane

Rockville, MD 20857

(800) 532-4440

(301) 827-4420

Web site: http://www.fda.gov

In Canada

Addictions Foundation of Manitoba

1031 Portage Avenue

Winnipeg, MB R3G 0R8

(204) 944-6200

Narcotics Anonymous (NA)

Help line: (416) 691-9519

They can refer you to a chapter in your area.

For Further Reading

Colvin, Rod. *Prescription Drug Abuse: The Hidden Epidemic*. Omaha, NE: Addicus Books, 1995.

Glass, George. *Drugs and Fitting In*. New York: Rosen Publishing Group, 1994.

Graedon, Joe, and Teresa Graedon. *The People's Guide to Deadly Drug Interactions*. New York: St. Martin's Press, 1998.

Ryan, Elizabeth A. *Straight Talk About Drugs and Alcohol*. New York: Facts on File, 1995.

Simpson, Carolyn. *RX: Reading and Following the Directions for All Kinds of Medications*. New York: Rosen Publishing Group, 1994.

Yoslow, Mark. *Drugs in the Body: Effects of Abuse*. New York: Franklin Watts, 1992.

Index

About the Author

Melanie Apel Gordon is a pediatric respiratory therapist at Children's Memorial Hospital in Chicago, Illinois. She has a bachelor's degree in respiratory care and another in theater arts. Melanie has written six children's books on health-related topics, and she is currently working on another six. She is also working on two books about cystic fibrosis. Melanie lives in Glenview, Illinois, with her husband Richard, dogs Fred and Ginger, and frogs Fluffy and Spike.

Photo Credits

Cover, pp. 21, 25 by John Bentham; pp. 10, 13, 23, 28, 32, 34, 38, 43, 45 by Ira Fox; p. 48 by Olga Palma; p. 55 by Brian T. Silak; p. 15 by Michael Brandt; p. 51 by Megan Alderson; p. 2 © Corbis/Ted Streshinsky; p. 8 © Corbis/Ed Eckstein, p.18 by Katie McClancy.